HOW TO USE TEA TREE OIL

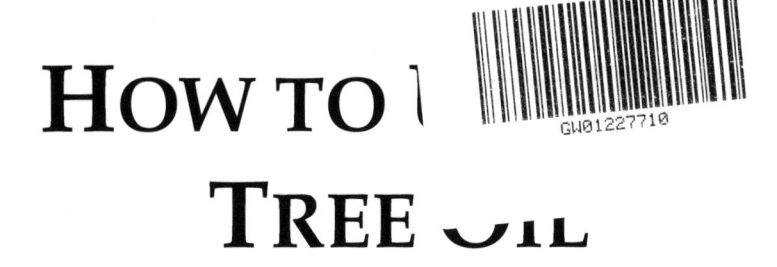

90 Great Ways to Use Natures "Medicine Cabinet in a Bottle"

RUTH ELSTON

BETTER LIFE BOOKS

Copyright © 2013 Ruth Elston
All rights reserved.
ISBN: 978-0-620-57246-0

To a healthy, natural life.

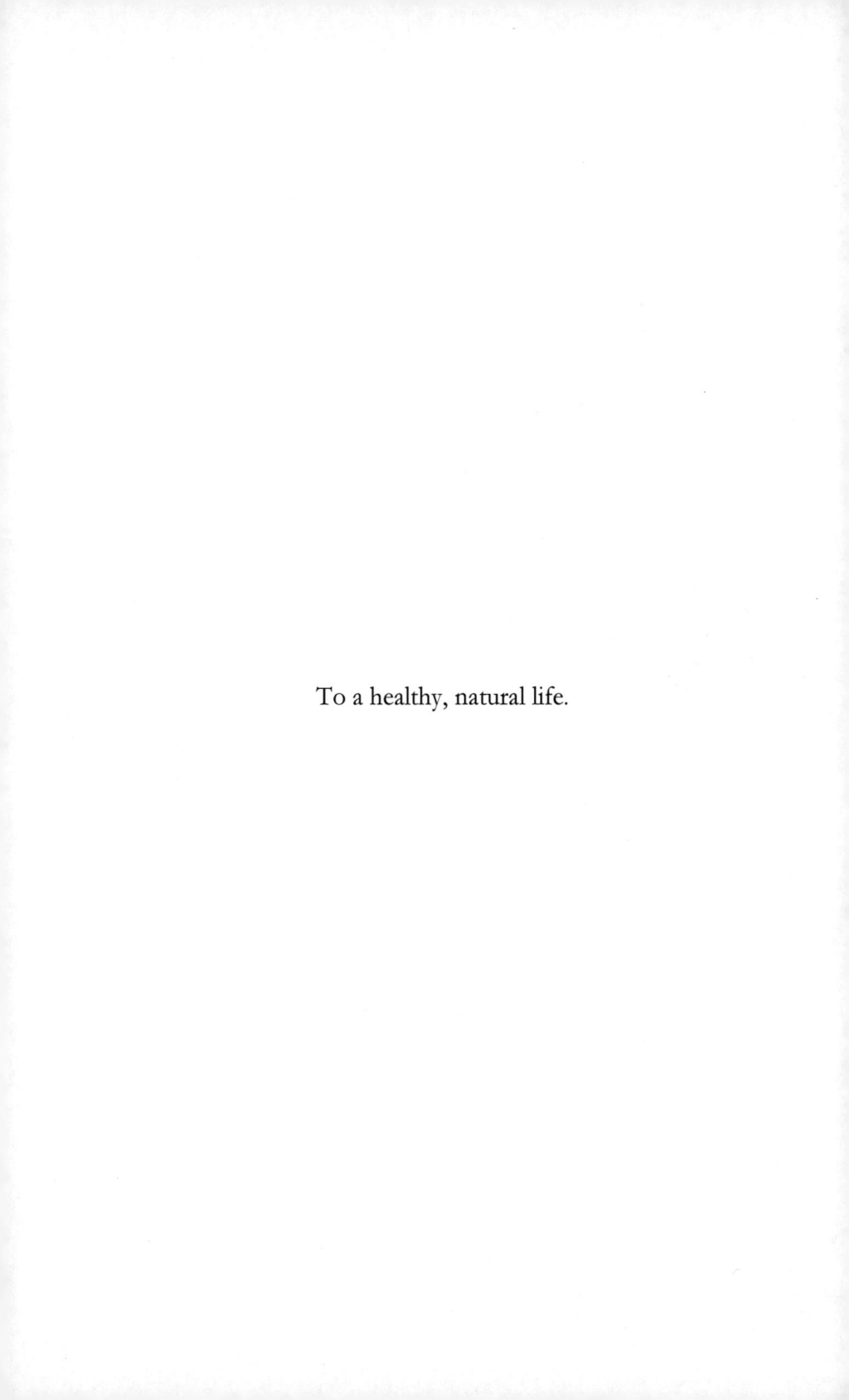

CONTENTS

INTRODUCTION 1
A IS FOR: ACNE, AIR FRESHENER AND ATHLETES FOOT 4
B IS FOR: BASE OILS, BLISTERS, BOILS, BUNIONS, BURNS & BURSITIS 11
C IS FOR: CANKER SORES, CARBUNCLES, CELL PHONE CLEANER, CHAPPED LIPS, CORNS & CALLUSES, COLD SORES AND CUTS & SCRAPES 16
D IS FOR: DANDRUFF AND DRY SKIN 25
E IS FOR: EAR INFECTIONS 28
F IS FOR: FACE MASK, FIRST AID AND FLEA CONTROL 30
G IS FOR: GUM REMOVER 33
H IS FOR: HALITOSIS, HAND WASH, HEAD LICE, HOUSEHOLD CLEANING AGENT AND HUMIDIFIERS 34
I IS FOR: INGROWN HAIRS, INSECT REPELLENT AND INSECT STINGS.43
L IS FOR: LARYNGITIS AND LEECHES 47
M IS FOR: MOUTHWASH 49
N IS FOR: NAIL FUNGUS 51
O IS FOR: OFFICE CLEANER 53
P IS FOR: PLANTAR WARTS, POOR CIRCULATION, POISON IVY AND PSORIASIS 55
R IS FOR: RINGWORM 60
S IS FOR: SHAVING, SINUS INFECTION, SLIVERS AND SPLINTERS, SKIN CARE, SPIDER SPRAY, SPRAINS AND SUNBURN 62
T IS FOR: TEA TREE SANITIZING WIPES AND TIRED FEET 67
U IS FOR: UNPLEASANT SMELLS 70
V IS FOR VAGINAL THRUSH 72
W IS FOR: WARTS AND WAXING 73
Y IS FOR: YOGA MATS 76
THE HISTORY OF TEA TREE OIL 77
STUDIES 79
MESSAGE FROM THE AUTHOR 82

ACKNOWLEDGMENTS

A big thank you to Tom at Better Life Books.

Also, to Lynne and Juanita for their help and suggestions.

Introduction

My publishers have called this 'A Complete Guide', but I'm not sure there is any such thing as 'complete' when it comes to the uses of Tea Tree oil. Almost every day I receive a story from someone who has found yet another way to successfully use the oil to help with an ailment or to put it to some other practical use.

Tea Tree oil has proven to be a powerful immune booster that sorts out most viral, bacterial and fungal infections in a snap. It is not only used by aromatherapists and herbalists, it is also widely used by the medical and veterinarian professions.

You can apply it to the skin for the treatment of fungal infections such as nail fungus, acne, athlete's foot, skin tags and ringworm. You can use it as an antiseptic for cuts and abrasions, burns, blisters, insect bites and stings, boils, vaginal infections, herpes, and minor wounds. The oil can be added to boiling water and the vapors will treat respiratory problems such as asthma, coughs, bronchitis, sore throats and pulmonary inflammation. When used as a mouth wash, it is very effective in healing fungal infections of the mouth and throat, as well as being helpful in easing toothache. By using Tea tree oil on the hair, scalp, combs and brushes, parents can completely eliminate head lice.

You can create your own natural cleaner that's both safe and effective for use throughout your home, office and even your car. You can add to your laundry wash loads that include diapers and pet blankets. Use on your garbage disposal to keep it clean, sanitized and fresh smelling. Tea Tree oil's multipurpose household spray disinfects items that can't go in with laundry, like mats, pillows and curtains. Or can be used in cupboards, on kitchen counters, cutting boards and in your refrigerator. Use in the bathroom on shower curtains and the seals around baths and showers. Clean your pet mat or litter boxes. It will help keep away ants, roaches, mosquitoes and get rid of your dog's fleas! In the office, use to clean and disinfect 'phones, keyboards and desktops.

Tea Tree oil can even be used to fight a number of infections that are resistant to antibiotics. It strengthens the body's immune system, which may have been weakened by the use of antibiotics and other drugs.
No home should ever be without this super "medicine cabinet in a bottle".

There are so many uses of Tea Tree oil; it can become a bit overwhelming. My purpose here is to offer some guidance on home remedies that have been successful for so many others and particularly ones that have proven so helpful in my household when other treatments failed.

In the remedies that follow you will learn how Tea Tree can be an even more effective when used in combination with other essential oils. Mixing with Lavender is one of my personal favorites. When you mix these two essential oils together you create a synergy that increases the power of both oils.

The following is an almost complete A - Z listing of how Tea Tree oil may best help you. Please do let me know if you have a favorite use for Tea Tree oil that I've missed.

A is for: Acne, Air Freshener and Athletes Foot

Acne

Acne is a skin disorder that appears as swellings, pimples and cysts, usually on the face. Although facial acne might cause the most concern, it is often more painful and harder to clear when it spreads to the chest, back and shoulders.

Most teenagers suffer from acne to some extent, and of course it can occur in adults as well. A severe acne outbreak can make teens very self conscious of their appearance.

Acne sufferers well know the frustration of searching for an acne product that really works. Maybe some of the products you've tried worked for a while, perhaps some didn't work at all and I'll bet others even made the problem worse. Studies have shown that Tea Tree oil offers a perfect alternative remedy for acne.

One study at the Department of Dermatology, Royal Prince Alfred Hospital in Camperdown, Australia, revealed Tea Tree oil's ability to perform just as well as any common over-the-counter acne treatment, but without the side effects. (SEE STUDIES AT END OF BOOK)

This scientific proof simply confirms the overwhelming anecdotal evidence built up by many thousands of users over many years of trial and error; Tea Tree oil works really well on acne and is kinder to your face than most other commercial treatments. It works by neutralizing the bacteria that causes pimples and acne to develop. The anti-bacterial properties kill the germs, they don't just deactivate them.

Using a soap that contains Tea Tree oil can be effective for those who have a mild form of acne, but the 100% pure Tea Tree oil is strongly recommended for severe cases. The oil can be applied directly to the pimple.

Janice, a nearby neighbor of mine, confessed to me that she was desperate to help her son Timothy find a solution for his acne. She felt it affected his self confidence and was making him very unhappy. She had taken him to the doctor and had bought various prescription and over-the-counter remedies but they were just not working.

Timothy had a severe form of acne which was painful and inflammatory. If not properly treated, this form of acne can take a month or two to heal and also lead to permanent acne scars.

I suggested that Timothy should try Tea Tree oil, as it had worked so well for my son during his teenage years.

Here is what Timothy told me about his experience:

"At first I was worried about putting oil on my skin because my skin was already quite oily. Sometimes the pimples on my cheeks hurt so much that I woke up in the middle of the night from pain. Anyway, after my mum told me you had recommended it I decided to give Tea Tree oil a try and I have to say wow - it works! I applied a drop on a cotton swab directly to each pimple. There was a slight stinging sensation when I applied the oil but then I noticed that the pimples didn't hurt anymore. I didn't like the smell but it disappeared as the oil dried. The next day the pimples were dry! Day by day my skin is definitely becoming clearer and the pimples aren't painful at all. Now every night I just mix Tea Tree oil with some water and apply it to my face. I've been using it for a couple of weeks and it's working well so far. Nothing else has ever worked for me like this has and I've tried many products. I must say, the oil has a strong scent so I wouldn't recommend applying it before going out on a date or anything, but my clear skin more than makes up for it. I'm certainly going to continue using and I've already told a few of my mates about it."

Once the condition is under control, there are two other natural products, Aloe Vera and Apple Cider Vinegar, both of which can be used to supplement the Tea Tree oil treatment.

Always test your skins sensitivity before using Tea Tree oil on your face. Put a couple drops of undiluted oil onto a cotton swab and then apply it to the inside of your forearm. Wait an hour or two and if there is no burning sensation and no rash has developed you can try a facial treatment.

If you do experience some irritation, dilute the oil: Start with five drops water - 5 drops oil and continue to re-test until you find a dilution that works for you.

Tea Tree oil is a fantastic anti-acne remedy but it works better when you give it some help and learn how to apply it correctly.

Clean skin is an absolute must before applying Tea Tree oil and the number one rule is to wash your face first. Use a Tea Tree Face Wash for deep cleaning. After washing your face, saturate a cotton swab with the Tea Tree oil solution that works for you. Apply this directly to the pimples, and leave it (no rinsing). Apply once in the morning and once at night.

Washing your face twice a day is a minimum requirement and at least once a day, use an astringent Tea Tree Rinse on your face. You make this by adding four drops of Tea Tree oil into a few cups of cold water.

Many people use the astringent rinse, or a commercial Tea Tree Face Wash, just to remain acne free and keep their skin glowing naturally.

There are other things you can do to help the Tea Tree oil clear your acne:

Hair on your forehead can cause pimples so consider changing your hairstyle thereby keeping hair away from your face.

Never dry your face on a towel you have used to dry your hair with and always dry your face using a clean fresh towel.

Avoid wiping perspiration from your face onto your sleeve (or any other cloth) when sweating profusely after exercise or playing sports. This can cause pimples by damaging the epidermis and introducing bacteria into the skin.

Tea Tree oil is a fantastic anti-acne remedy, but it works even better when you give it some help!

Air Freshener

How "Fresh" Is Your Air Freshener?

According to Time Magazine (article by Coco Masters, Sept. 24, 2007), not very!

Many chemical air fresheners are just not nice to the body or the environment and are a particular problem for people with allergies and chemical sensitivities. The Time Magazine article reported that many air fresheners they tested contain phthalates, a chemical banned in many countries.

So, when opening your windows just isn't enough, Tea Tree oil offers a great natural alternative to these potential health hazards.

Just mix 1 teaspoon of Tea Tree oil with 1 cup of water,

add to a spray bottle and you have a marvelous, all natural air freshener. I like to add a few drops of Lavender or some lemon juice to this mixture, especially for a nice bathroom spray.

Another simple alternative is to add a few drops of Tea Tree oil and Lavender oil to the water of a humidifier to permeate and purify the surrounding air.

(SEE CHAPTER ON UNPLEASANT SMELLS)

Athlete's Foot

Athlete's Foot is a fungal growth on the skin of the foot that causes peeling, redness, itching, and burning between the toes. Its medical term is Tinea pedis. It can also occur between the fingers, and in the groin area (Jock Itch). The condition is highly contagious, and thrives in warm, moist areas. It is passed through contact with items such as shoes, stockings, and in shower or pool surfaces.

Athlete's Foot infections range from mild to severe and may last just a few days, or for several weeks. Fortunately, the condition always responds well to Tea

Tree oil's powerful anti-fungal properties! However, if proper preventative measures are not in place it could return.

To treat Athlete's Foot, just saturate a cotton swab with Tea Tree oil and apply directly to the affected and surrounding area. Do this at least twice a day, preferably morning and night.

PREVENTION IS BETTER THAN CURE!

To prevent Athlete's Foot, follow these measures:

> Wash your feet with soap and water, preferably twice a day.
> Always dry your feet carefully, but thoroughly, with your own clean towel. Never share towels.
> Wear clean, natural fiber (cotton or wool) socks and change them often.
> Wear well ventilated leather shoes.
> Wear sandals or flip-flops at a public showers, locker rooms and pools.
> Keep your own tub or shower clean.

"The bottom line is your feet are teeming with fungal diversity, so wear your flip flops in locker rooms if you don't want to mix your foot fungi with someone else's fungi" Dr Julia Segre - National Institutes of Health, USA.

Tea Tree oil is also effective for other fungal skin infections such as Jock Itch (SEE LATER CHAPTER ON RINGWORM)

B is for: Base Oils, Blisters, Boils, Bunions, Burns & Bursitis

Base Oils (Carriers)

You can dilute Tea Tree oil with base oils (sometimes called carrier oils). There is a wide variety of oils that can be used for this purpose but I find I use Avocado, Olive and Almond oils the most often. These are some other base oils that are used:

Apricot Kernel oil - Coconut oil - Cranberry Seed oil - Evening Primrose oil - Grapeseed oil - Hemp Seed oil - Rose Hip oil - Sesame oil - Sunflower oil - Watermelon Seed oil.

Aromaweb has everything you would ever need to know about base/carrier oils. You can find them at *aromaweb.com*

For insect bites, cuts and grazes, burns and sunburn a 10 percent concentration is an appropriate mixture of Tea Tree oil with base oil. Mix 1 tablespoon of Tea Tree oil to a half cup of base oil.

A stronger mixture is more suitable for anti-fungal treatments. Mix 2 tablespoon of Tea Tree oil to half a cup of base oil and this will give you a twenty percent concentration.

For pain and inflammation associated with bruises, bunions, bursitis, eczema, gout, and sprains, it is usually best to use a mix Tea Tree oil with an Arnica gel at between 5 -10 percent concentration.

Blisters

Working in the garden or walking in ill-fitting new shoes - just two of the many ways you can end up with painful blisters. Any type of friction on the skin can result in a blister, which means the most common places they occur are on the feet and hands.

Tea Tree oil's natural antiseptic properties dry out the blister and help it heal more quickly. Wash the area around the blister and treat with a few drops of undiluted Tea Tree oil.

Boils

Tea Tree oil can be applied undiluted to boils, but first make a skin wash using diluted Tea Tree oil. For this, use one cup of warm water and add 5 drops of Tea Tree oil.

Make sure to wash the area around the boil thoroughly and then use a cotton bud to apply full strength Tea Tree oil direct to the boil. You can tape a gauze pad saturated with diluted oil directly to the boil for up to twelve hours. (Use a dilution that works for your skin type)

To avoid any contamination dispose of all the old gauze or cotton balls after each treatment and remember to always wash your hands!

Bunions

Bunions present alongside your big toe. Most bunions are caused by shoes with too tight a point that pushes your toes to a point (which is why ballet dancers suffer bunions). Wearing high-heeled shoes often causes bunions.

As a good treatment for bunions, try soaking the foot in a mixture of one tablespoon of Tea Tree oil, two tablespoons of Epsom salts and six cups of hot water.

Burns

Tea Tree oil is excellent for burns but speedy treatment is essential. The burn area should be flushed immediately with cold water, or packed with ice if possible. If the burn area is too sensitive for the oil to be applied by a finger or cotton bud, apply liberally direct from the bottle. The cold water and Tea Tree oil treatment can be alternated every 5-10 minutes. The oil can also safely be applied to any blistering..

Self treatment is only appropriate for 1st and 2nd degree burns - you should seek medical assistance urgently for anything more serious. In all instances, Arnica will help relieve any associated shock.

Bursitis

Bursitis is as an inflammation or irritation which affects the various joints of the body. It is a painful condition that has a variety of causes. Without the help of a medical professional it's hard to tell the difference between bursitis and pain caused by a strain or arthritis.

Depending on the cause, in many cases Tea Tree oil remedies can be used instead of prescription pain relievers. Bacterial infections sometimes cause bursitis, in which cases Tea Tree oil is most appropriate. For bursitis occurring after traumatic injury or strain, Tea Tree oil mixed with an Arnica gel and applied to the affected area provides excellent short-term pain relief. Apply ice packs, before and after applying the gel.

C is for: Canker Sores, Carbuncles, Cell Phone Cleaner, Chapped Lips, Corns & Calluses, Cold Sores and Cuts & Scrapes

Canker Sores

Canker sores, also known as mouth ulcers, can form on the gums, inner cheeks and lips. The sores may form from pinhead size to lesions the size of a shirt button, and can be very painful. Canker sores usually appear on the inner surface of the cheeks and lips, tongue, soft palate, and the base of the gums. They are a localized bacterial infection characterized by one or more painful, red spots or a bump that develops into an open ulcer. They originate from a variety of causes such as, biting your cheek, wearing dentures, and even eating hard foods. Children wearing braces often develop Canker sores.

Anyone can develop a canker sore but for some reason women are more likely to get them than men. It seems that Canker sores may run in families.

At the first sign of a canker sore, apply a 50/50 diluted Tea Tree oil to the sore. Use a cotton swab to apply the mixture directly to the canker sore. Repeat the treatment three to four times a day. Rinsing with a Tea Tree oil mouthwash will also help reduce the symptoms: (See Mouthwash)

Carbuncles

A carbuncle is an abscess similar to a boil, but bigger. The infected area usually has one or more openings draining pus onto the skin. This painful condition is also caused by the staphylococcus organism. The presence of carbuncles can actually be seen as a sign that the immune system is working, but that doesn't make the condition any easier to live with

Carbuncles may develop anywhere, but they are most

common on the back and the neck. They may be red and irritated, and might hurt when touched. They may also grow very fast and have a white or yellow center. Healing usually takes longer than when treating boils and they can be more difficult to cure.

Carbuncles can be caused by various factors that are often difficult to determine. The infection is contagious and poor hygiene, poor nutrition or weakening of the immune system, can make you vulnerable. It is known that persons with diabetes and immune system diseases are more likely to develop bacterial infections.

Carbuncles usually must drain before they will heal. If left untreated, within two weeks the immune system ramps up its repulsion of the bacteria. Treatment by a health professional is certainly needed if the carbuncle lasts longer than two weeks, or returns frequently.

It is important to refrain from squeezing them as squeezing causes more pain and also increases the risk of spreading the infection This often happens when the carbuncle is on the buttocks or back where it may get squashed and cause the fluids inside to burst.

To treat a carbuncle at home, you can apply a warm compresses soaked in a mixture of 10 drops of Tea Tree oil per cup of very warm water to the area for 30 minutes. The warmth will open up the blood vessels, helping it to drain and relieve the pain. Apply 3-4 times a day and let dry naturally. The Tea Tree Oil acts like an antiseptic and will help heal as well as stop the infection spreading. Crushed garlic or Manuka Honey on the carbuncle beneath the hot compress can help draw out the pus. Keep the carbuncle clean and dry between compress treatments. If possible, do not cover it with clothing.

A warm Tea Tree oil bath will help bring a carbuncle to a head in hard-to-reach places such as the back, groin or buttocks.

Use a clean washcloth each time, and be sure that no one else uses those cloths. Proper hygiene is very important to prevent the spread of infection. After treating a carbuncle, hands should always be washed thoroughly with a Tea Tree oil soap or your own Tea Tree oil rinse. Washcloths and towels must not be shared or reused. Clothing, washcloths, towels, and sheets or other items that contact infected areas should be washed in very hot water that includes at least 10 drops of Tea Tree oil.

PREVENTION OF CARBUNCLES

As previously mentioned the infection is contagious and may spread to other areas of the body, or to other people living in the same residence. Once a person has experienced carbuncles, they can frequently recur. There are several ways prevent re-infection. These include:

>   Good personal hygiene.
>   Good hand-washing techniques
>   The use of Tea Tree oil products

Also, strengthen your immune system by drinking Echinacea tea, plenty of water and eating properly.

Cell Phone Cleaner

"Now hear this! Your cellphone is as dirty as a toilet seat - even the bottom of your shoe" writes the New York Post (CYNTHIA R. FAGEN , August 3, 2006)

Quoting microbiologist professor Joanna Verran the New York Post warns mobile phone users that the combination of constant handling and the heat generated by the phone can cause pimples and boils, even meningitis and pneumonia. Bacteria thrive under these conditions and the cell phone contains more skin bacteria than any other object.

Tea Tree oil cleansing wipes are naturally anti-bacterial and there are several commercial products available that you could use. However, you don't want to get water damage to your cell phone during the cleaning process, or scratch the screen and a few drops of Tea Tree oil on a tissue or piece of cotton is more than enough to clean your cell phone and rid it of all those nasty germs.

Chapped Lips

The main cause of chapped lips is dehydration and exposure to the elements. Try not to constantly lick or pick at them or you'll only make matters worse.

Clear away any dead skin by gently rubbing a soft cloth (or a Tea Tree Oil Sanitizing Wipe) along your lips. Then apply a Tea Tree oil lip balm, or just add a few drops of Tea Tree oil to your favorite moisturizer or salve and use that.

There are many recipes for making your own lip balm on the web, using beeswax etc. They seem a bit complicated to me, but if you do decide to make your own do include Tea Tree Oil and Coconut Oil.

Prevention is better than cure

Drink more water! It's not just your lips that will thank you. By drinking more water, you are helping your skin all around, boosting your skin in the fight against the aging process. Use a lip sun block when you spend any excessive time outdoors.

Cold Sores

Cold Sores are caused by the herpes simplex 1 virus, which most of us pick up as children. A study by Dr Christine Carson and her colleagues at The University of Western Australia shows that Tea Tree oil has significant anti-viral activity against the herpes simplex virus.

When the virus is activated, cold sores usually appear on the mouth or lips. Normally, they tend to disappear naturally after about seven to ten days.

Although 25 to 40 per cent of people are prone to developing cold sores, there is still no cure for them. However, there is also nothing better than using Tea Tree oil for limiting the pain and duration of these sores.

Take these steps to treat the sore at the first sign of an outbreak:

1. Apply an ice cube to the cold sore for a few minutes as this will ease the pain and reduce the chances of the sore spreading.

2. Wash the cold sore area using a Tea Tree Face Wash.

You can make your own face cleansing wash by adding four drops of Tea Tree oil to one cup of hot water.

3. Put two or three drops of undiluted Tea Tree oil on a Q-tip or cotton bud and apply it directly to the cold sore. Try not to get undiluted oil onto your healthy skin; using petroleum jelly around the area of the sore will be helpful.

Repeat twice a day.

Use Tea Tree oil carefully and remember it is powerful, so don't apply it too often or you'll end up with a raw spot on your skin. You can apply petroleum jelly to the area surrounding the Cold Sore to protect the healthy skin.

Corns & Calluses

Corns usually appear on the tops of your toes and they are often caused by friction from a pair of ill fitting shoes. My sister swears they are more painful in cold weather!

A Tea Tree oil soak will soften corns and calluses. Use a mixture of one teaspoon of Tea Tree oil, two tablespoons of Epsom salts and six cups of hot water.

Soak the feet for at least 5 minutes. A teaspoon of Apple Cider Vinegar or lemon juice can also be added.

Try to give the feet a soak at least 3 times a day, but if this isn't possible dab the corns with Tea Tree oil (use cotton wool or bud) as often as you can.

Cuts & Scrapes

The first thing you need to do is to clean and disinfect the area to prevent infection. Wash the wound and surrounding areas with diluted Tea Tree oil but you can apply undiluted direct to the cut.

Cuts and scrapes heal more quickly with an application of Tea Tree oil. Leave uncovered if possible, but with children it is better to cover the cut with a band aid to ensure they don't get oil on their fingers and into their mouths.

D is for: Dandruff and Dry Skin

Dandruff

Persistent itching and flaking are the hallmark signs of Dandruff. Studies have shown the use of 5% Tea Tree Shampoo significantly reduces these symptoms.

Shampooing with Tea Tree oil cleans the hair and helps to reduce the bacteria that cause Dandruff. A Tea Tree Shampoo also protects the hair from physical damage and generally improves resistance to harmful influences of the environment. Best results are achieved by regular use.

You can use specialty shampoos that have Tea Tree oil blended in and are ready to use right out of the bottle, or you can add a few drops of Tea Tree oil to your regular shampoo.

To use your own mixture, simply pour a small amount

of shampoo in your palm and add a few drops of Tea Tree oil and then massage into your scalp. Using too much oil can reduce the amount of suds from your shampoo, so you might have to adjust the amount of Tea Tree oil accordingly.

Leave the mixture in your hair for 3 to 4 minutes before rinsing off.

When using your own mixture you will experience a cool and tingling sensation on your scalp. If you experience more of a burning sensation rinse off at once and use a weaker mixture next time.

You may have to follow this routine for a week or two before seeing consistent results.

I use this mixture whenever I want to give my hair and scalp a really good deep-cleaning.

Dry Skin

There are many wonderful Tea Tree Moisturizers available, but if you want to make your own just mix a few drops of Tea Tree oil with a carrier oil of your choice (Almond oil, Aloe Vera or Coconut oil would be good choices). Try blending your own mixture with oils and creams that work for you. Aim for a moisturizer that is light and milky, and that spreads and dissolves into your skin easily.

A Tea Tree Moisturizer is the perfect companion for the Tea Tree Face Wash and will soothe and heal dry skin.

I find a moisturizer fortified with Tea Tree oil and Aloe Vera helps to soothe, restore and maintain the soft feel I love in my skin.

.

E is for: Ear Infections

Ear Infections

Tea Tree oil is a natural alternative to antibiotics for healing Ear Infections, but undiluted Tea Tree oil must never be used directly into the ear!

I cannot emphasize this too strongly; Tea Tree oil is a powerful essential oil that can burn and you must dilute it. For ear infections you should dilute with good quality base oil - Olive, Almond etc. Do not dilute with water as this will only aggravate the infection.

Any remedy placed inside the ear should first be warmed to a comfortable temperature.

Tea Tree oil with Olive oil

Mix 1 drop of Tea Tree oil to 1 tablespoon of warm Olive oil and pour 3 drops of this mixture into the ear with the help of a dropper; or trickle a small amount into the ear as needed. Then put a ball of cotton wool into your ear.

Use this mixture twice a day with one treatment at bedtime. The mixture can also be rubbed on the back of the ear to help relieve pain.

Garlic oil, or juice, is another natural remedy that helps fight ear infection and can be added to the Tea Tree oil & Olive oil mixture.

If you suspect the earache is anything other than an infection i.e. a punctured or ruptured eardrum, do not home treat with any home remedy but rather consult a doctor.

F is for: Face Mask, First Aid and Flea Control

Face Mask

A mixture of Tea Tree oil, Carrot Seed oil (just a few drops of each) and a small amount of plain yoghurt makes a refreshing face mask. Leave this on your face for as long as is comfortable (at least 10 minutes) before rinsing off.

Another indulgent recipe that helps remove blemishes: Tea Tree oil, Aloe Vera, Manuka Honey (if you can get it, if not use plain honey), sea salt, plain Greek yogurt, Apple Cider vinegar, and baking soda.

First-Aid

Dr. Philip Tierno, author of The Secret Life of Germs believes that all families should prepare a first aid kit with supplies to cope with everyday emergencies such as cuts and scrapes. His very sensible suggestions for what should be in your first aid kit includes; gauze wraps and pads, butterfly tape that can be used as a stitch, scissors, bandages, a splint or board in case someone breaks a bone, a first-aid manual, eye wash and eye pad, instant ice packs, anti-bacterial ointment, latex gloves, Tea Tree oil (for infections, cuts and abrasions), aspirin, ibuprofen, and vitamin supplements. To this I would add Tea Tree Anti-bacterial Ointment, Tea Tree Sanitizing Wipes and at least one bottle of Arnica.

Flea Control

Tea Tree oil is especially useful for repelling fleas in dogs but do not use Tea Tree oil on your cats as their skin is far too sensitive for it. You must use Tea Tree oil regularly to prevent fleas from attaching to the dog.

There are three good ways to prevent flea infestation;

>A Tea Tree oil "Flea Collar".
>Bathing your dog with Tea Tree oil shampoo.
>Spraying your dog with a Tea Tree oil mist.

To make a flea collar with Tea Tree oil, simply pour a few drops of undiluted Tea Tree oil on the dog's regular collar and repeat every second week.

There are dog shampoos available that include Tea Tree oil but you can self treat if you prefer. After bathing your dog with its regular shampoo, just add Tea Tree oil to the rinse water. A few drops will be enough, depending on the size of your dog. It is preferable to let the dog air dry.

To make a spray for your dog, mix 6 drops of Tea Tree oil with 3 cups of water in a spray bottle and mix vigorously. Brush your dog's fur in the wrong direction and spray its coat with this water/Tea Tree oil mist every second day. Make sure to avoid the eyes!

Prevention is always better than cure and as mentioned in an earlier chapter you should wash all of your dogs bedding and day blankets in the washing machine after adding a few drops of Tea Tree oil.

Please remember, Tea Tree oil is not suitable for cats!

G is for: Gum Remover

Gum Remover

I accidentally sat on bubble gum at a schools sport event and didn't notice until I got into the car on the way home. Undiluted Tea Tree oil removed to gum from my skirt and the car seat! My husband was slightly concerned about using full strength Tea Tree oil on his car upholstery but it didn't hurt the surface at all and it took the gum right off.

Pour full strength Tea Tree oil on an old towel or piece of cloth and then lightly dab the gum area. After about a minute, rub to loosen the gum and then wash the item after adding a few drops of Tea Tree oil to your normal detergent.

H is for: Halitosis, Hand Wash, Head Lice, Household Cleaning Agent and Humidifiers

Halitosis

Tea Tree oil is an excellent remedy for halitosis. These days you can buy a whole range of Tea Tree oil products to combat bad breath including: Toothpastes, mouthwashes, chewing sticks, oil infused toothpicks and even Tea Tree Mouth Sprays.

Why is Tea Tree oil so useful in combating halitosis? Well, Bacteria in your mouth are the principal causes of mouth odor and Tea Tree Oil's antiseptic qualities kill the fungi and bacteria that feed on food particles left in the mouth. Tests on 162 different oral bacteria by the Tea Tree Oil Research Group at University of Western Australia showed that all were killed by concentrations of 2% Tea Tree oil.

Tea Tree oil must be diluted before using in the mouth. As with all mouthwashes, care should be taken not to swallow when using Tea Tree oil.

When used as part of your routine mouth care, Tea Tree oil not only kills the bacteria that causes bad breath, but it is also helps the fight against oral candidiasis, gingivitis, inflamed gums, mouth sores and ulcers.

By far the best way to use Tea Tree oil for bad breath is to start a proper dental care program and stick to it. It will only take a few extra minutes a day to get a good routine going. The perfect plan to eliminate bad breath is to brush your teeth with a Tea Tree oil toothpaste at least twice a day and follow this by flossing between your teeth. You can then freshen your breath on the go with a Tea Tree oil mouthwash.

You can also keep your toothbrush germ-free by soaking it in a solution of 5-10 drops of Tea Tree Oil in a cup of water for about ten minutes or so.

When it comes to using Tea Tree oil in the mouth I recommend using propriety brand products that have been made for the specific purpose. If you prefer to make your own mouthwash a solution of 2 drops Tea Tree oil to about a half cup of warm water should suffice.

Hand Wash

It's a sad fact that even in these modern times, most people don't wash their hands either often enough or well enough. New research suggests fecal matter can be found on more than a quarter of our hands, and often the quantity of germs is equivalent to the number in a dirty toilet bowl!

Many hospitals now routinely use Tea Tree oil products for hand washing after scientific studies revealed them to be effective in eliminating bacteria. A study published in the Journal of Hospital Infection in 2005 showed that Tea Tree oil formulations helped reduce hospital-acquired infections such as those caused by Staphylococcus aureus, or 'golden staph'.

Tea Tree oil also makes a wonderful anti-bacterial hand wash in the home. To make your own, just add a few drops to any liquid soap. I always carry Tea Tree Sanitizing Wipes for all those occasions where proper hand washing facilities aren't available.

Head Lice

Head Lice is such a serious problem that the subject deserves a book of its own rather than just this chapter concerning how Tea Tree oil can help with their control.

According to The Lice Ladies (Joan Sawyer and Roberta MacPhee) in their award winning video Head Lice to Dead Lice, Head Lice cause serious stress to more than 15 million American families a year. Millions of children are missing critical days of school work because they cannot get rid of head lice.

The Lice Ladies extol a simple natural way you can get rid of head lice by smothering them with olive oil. But you need to know how to do it right. It's not just a case of dumping olive oil on the head and praying. They need smothering, and smothering head lice is a process. Female adult lice lay eggs every day, so that each day a new generation hatches on the head. Therefore, the infested head must be treated correctly with olive oil at specific times over the 21-day life cycle of the louse in order to kill each generation at its most vulnerable stage, and before it is old enough to lay eggs of its own. Using the olive oil method you will no longer waste your money on expensive and ineffective chemicals. Save your money and get on with your life. I promise you, it works.

Tea Tree oil is the perfect natural product to support the olive oil method and ensure that the lice are not just killed but the whole infestation controlled so that their eggs do not re-infect and spread. By using Tea Tree oil on the hair, scalp, combs, brushes, pillowcases and anything else that comes into contact with the lice you will be able to eliminate the little critters completely

Apply undiluted Tea Tree oil to the scalp (or at least as strong a dilution as the skin can tolerate) - leave this for 30 minutes and then wash the hair. Use a Tea Tree Shampoo regularly. (See chapter on Dandruff.)

Lice and their eggs may get onto pillow cases, towels and other fabrics, so add 20 drops Tea Tree oil to the washing.

Combs, brushes and hair clippers should also be disinfected and cleansed with a Tea Tree oil solution. Soak non electrical items in a mixture of 10 drops of Tea Tree oil per cup of very warm water (See chapter on Cleaning)

Household Cleaning Agent

Tea Tree oil is anti-bacterial and antimicrobial making it the perfect all natural cleaning agent for your home. It's easy to create your own natural cleaner that's both safe and effective.

If you have been suffering from any of the fungal infections mentioned in this book it would be a good idea to add Tea Tree oil to your laundry wash. Add one teaspoonful to the detergent in the washing machine to deep clean your laundry. This will combat recurrences of infections that can be transferred from towels, underwear, socks etc.

It's also a good idea to add a few drops of Tea Tree oil to wash loads that include diapers and pet blankets.

"Always the dirtiest thing by far is the kitchen sponge," says John Oxford, professor of virology at the University of London and chair of the Hygiene Council - an international body that compares hygiene standards across the world. Its latest study examined samples from homes in nine different countries, and found that more than 2o% of "visibly clean" kitchen cloths actually have high levels of contamination. The cloths also fail the bacterial test which looks for E.coli. Beware also of dust rags, dishrags, mops and other cleaning tools. Unless sanitized with Tea Tree Oil between uses, they only spread around the germs you are trying to kill

It is therefore essential to add Tea Tree oil when

cleaning these items.

Pour a little undiluted Tea Tree oil down your garbage disposal to keep it clean, sanitized and fresh smelling.

For a very effective multipurpose household spray, simply mix 2 teaspoons Tea Tree oil, 3 tablespoons Cider vinegar, and 2 cups of water together in a spray bottle.

You can use this to spray on items that can't go in with laundry, like mats, pillows and curtains.

Spray the same mixture into cupboards, on kitchen counters, cutting boards and other surfaces; then wipe clean. Dr Chuck Gerba, professor of microbiology at the University of Arizona says there are about 200 times more fecal bacteria on the average cutting board than on a toilet seat! This comes from the fecal bacteria in raw meat products. Tea Tree oil kills such bacteria stone dead!

Don't forget the refrigerator - more than 40% of fridge interiors failed 'Hygiene in the Home' tests on bacteria and mold build-up

To prevent mold and mildew in the bathroom; spray on the walls and ceiling above the shower and on surfaces like the shower curtain. Pay particular attention to the seals around baths and showers where 'Hygiene in the Home Studies' show 70% fail bacterial tests.

Spray onto a soft cloth and use to wipe your telephone to clean and disinfect, naturally.

This combination of natural products makes a powerful

disinfectant and can also be used to clean your pet mat or litter boxes. It will help keep away ants, fleas, roaches and other creepy crawlies.

You can use this same mixture for all areas of the home that need some help; airing out cupboards that are rarely used, suitcases that have been stored away or wherever there is a stale-smelling mustiness. (SEE CHAPTER ON UNPLEASANT SMELLS)

Humidifiers

I'm a big fan of humidifiers; we have a large one for the whole house and small ones in all of the bedrooms. We let them run 24/7 during the winter months. We originally bought humidifiers on the advice of my pediatrician who suggested that they would help with sinus infections/coughs etc.

However, you have to be careful because doctors also say humidifiers can spread germs and mold. "You can imagine in a humidifier that has all those bacteria, those molds that may be growing as well, and what you're doing is you're dispersing them into the air," Dr. Erwin Gelfand, chairman of the Department of Pediatrics at National Jewish Health, said in a recent NPR interview.

I put Tea Tree oil in mine and don't have any problems with bacteria growth. If I didn't add Tea Tree oil, they could get gross pretty quickly. I put just 10-15 drops in the whole house one once a week and 3-5 drops in the bedroom units. It smells so clean too. (SEE AIR FRESHENER)

I is for: Ingrown Hairs, Insect Repellent and Insect Stings

Ingrown Hairs

Ingrown hair is a condition where hair curls back and grows into the skin. They can affect the face, neck, legs, or any part of the body, but more commonly in areas that are shaved regularly. You only really need Tea Tree oil if they become infected. The Symptoms will include a rash and itching, burning skin.

Add a few drops of Tea Tree oil to a cup of very hot water and use it to soak a washcloth. Wring it out slightly, and press it against the ingrown hair. Repeat as necessary this treatment will soften the hair and bring it closer to the surface.

Adding Tea Tree oil to an Aloe Vera or Arnica gel can help prevent Ingrown Hairs. After shaving, gently massage the gel onto the shaved area.

Insect Repellent

Tea Tree oil is a great natural mosquito and insect repellent and is known to repel most insects that bite. There are two different preparations you will need, one to repel insects from your home and another that can be applied to your body.

Add 12 drops of Tea Tree oil to a pint of water in a misting spray bottle. Spray this natural bug buster to any areas where insects are prone. You can also spray the same mixture on your clothes when outdoors or camping.

My friend Sally keeps the insects away from her house by spraying Tea Tree oil on pieces of cloth and hanging them near windows and doors. I like dropping Tea Tree oil on candles and find this works particularly well.

There is no exact recipe for Tea Tree oil insect repellent that can be used on your body, but what you will need is full strength Tea Tree oil and a base/carrier oil. In this instance, I prefer to use Coconut oil as my base oil, but you can just as well use Jojoba, Almond oil, vegetable oil or even baby oil. Just add a few drops of Tea Tree oil to the base oil of your choice and rub on exposed skin.

Other essential oils that work well as insect repellents are Citronella, Cinnamon, Peppermint, and Lavender. You can add one or two of these with Tea Tree oil and mix with your chosen base oil. I'm sure there are other ones as well, but remember whichever essential oils you use, always dilute with a base oil. Mix well, apply!
(SEE CHAPTER ON BASE OILS)

Insect Bites & Stings

If you do get stung and the bite or sting threatens to become infected, then Tea Tree oil is a very useful natural home remedy to have around. It sterilizes and kills harmful bacteria that can get underneath the skin through insect bites and stings.

It's best to wash around the affected area with diluted Tea Tree oil and then apply undiluted Tea Tree oil directly to the bite or sting with your finger or cotton ball as soon as possible. (After you have removed any stinger that's been left behind)

Tea Tree oil will usually stop the itch and reduce any swelling very quickly, but you may have to apply it a few times a day before the bite or sting is completely healed.

L is for: Laryngitis and Leeches

Laryngitis

Bacterial infections are often the cause of laryngitis i.e. the common cold, flu, and bronchitis. These put strain on the vocal cords. Very occasionally it occurs due to fungal infection when your immune system is running low. In all these cases Tea Tree oil can help.

A Tea Tree oil gargle is an effective remedy for clearing up laryngitis. Using a cup of lukewarm water, add four drops of Tea Tree oil along with 1 tsp. of salt and stir well. Gargle 3 or 4 times a day.

A Tea Tree Mouthwash (see Mouthwash chapter) and Tea Tree Lozenges are also helpful.

Leeches

Apply undiluted Tea Tree oil directly to the live leech and leave it on for about 20 minutes or until the leech drops off. An application of Tea Tree Bug Spray will help avoid leeches. (See chapter on Insect Repellent)

M is for: Mouthwash

Mouthwash

The mouth harbors many unfriendly germs and Tea Tree oil's anti-bacterial properties make it a perfect solution for problems such as gingivitis and mouth sores. Researchers at Zürich University have clearly demonstrated that Tea Tree oil reduces the oral bacteria that can cause tooth decay, gingivitis, mouth ulcers and bad breath.

As a daily preventive measure, in addition to your normal oral hygiene routine, it is more than enough to simply add 1 drop of Tea Tree oil to a half cup of water and gargle. In fact you could just add 1 drop to the mouthwash that you currently use.

My daughter Jenny, makes her own Tea Tree Mouthwash and she prefers to add peppermint. This is her simple recipe:

3 cups of water (Jenny uses mineral water)
8 drops of Peppermint oil
8 drops of Tea-tree oil

When using Tea Tree oil mouthwash to fight gum infections (gingivitis), mouth ulcers, throat infections and tonsillitis you need a stronger dilution.

As with all mouthwashes, do not swallow!

Use a Tea Tree oil mouthwash and your mouth will thank you!

N is for: Nail Fungus

Nail Fungus

Tea Tree oil will clear up Nail Fungus on both toenails and fingernails, but results vary from person to person and stubborn infections can take several months to clear.

Nail Fungus, also known as onychomycosis, is quite a common nail infection which affects an estimated 5% of the population. It is in many ways similar to Athlete's Foot, and thrives in the same damp public areas, such as locker rooms, showers, etc. It can be very difficult to treat and can often last for 6 months to a year.

The most common symptom of Nail Fungus is the nail becoming thickened and discolored. Fungal infections of the nails appear as white, black, yellow or green dots underneath the nail. Toenails are more vulnerable to the infection than fingernails.

People are more prone to Nail Fungus if they have a history of athlete's foot. Diabetics and anyone with a weakened immune system are also more at risk. Nail Fungus is more common in men and older adults.

To treat the condition with Tea Tree oil, trim your nail back and apply 100% pure Tea Tree oil with a cotton bud or soft toothbrush two or three times a day. Apply it above and under the tip of the nail. Continue to apply the oil until the new nail has completely re-grown. Be patient, in most cases this is a long term treatment.

Some time ago, Julie, a neighbor of mine, showed me her Nail Fungus that she had been hiding behind nail paint until the nail starting coming away from the nail bed. I recommended she try Tea Tree oil and this is what she told me recently:

"I've suffered from Nail Fungus for longer than I care to remember and it was getting so bad that half the nail started coming loose. I had to paint the nail to hide the fungus and could only hope it wouldn't spread to other nails.
Then you told me about Tea Tree oil. As you suggested, I bought the 100% pure oil. I cut away the part of the nail that had lifted away from the skin and then applied the oil as you instructed. Then every night, I rubbed the Tea Tree oil into the affected area. The undiluted Tea Tree oil did cause some irritation as you said it might, but nothing too severe. Having used the oil for over a month now, my nail is growing back and it seems perfect. I really do see my nail problem coming to an end. Amazing - After all this time, no more fungus! I can't believe that I've spent all that money, and wasted all that time, when all I needed was simple natural oil. Thank you Ruth - IT WORKS!"

SEE THE CHAPTER ON ATHLETE'S FOOT FOR SOME ADDITIONAL PREVENTION TIPS

O is for: Office Cleaner

Office Cleaner

"Keyboards can carry more than 200 times as many bacteria as a toilet seat," **according to USA Today.**

"Which? Magazine found that the keyboards at its London offices contained up to five times more germs than a toilet seat," reports the London Daily Mail.

Dr Chuck Gerba , professor of microbiology at the University of Arizona, studies how diseases are transferred through the environment. This involves swabbing everyday items and measuring how many bacteria - and what sort - develops.

He particularly looks for fecal bacteria such as Staphylococcus aureus, or 'golden staph' as this superbug is also known. Dr Gerba says the office is a particularly bad source of germs. *"The average desktop has 400 times more bacteria than on a toilet seat"*, he says.

Tea Tree Sanitizing Wipes are especially useful in the office where you can't be sure what the cleaning staff have or haven't cleaned, or how they cleaned it. Use them for your 'phone, desktop, keyboard, laptop and anywhere else you think germs may thrive. Drawers in your desk where you might keep your lunchbox should be wiped regularly.

Not only will your own health be better protected but you will also reduce the risk of taking germs home to your loved ones. So don't forget to use Tea Tree Sanitizing Wipes on anything you transport between home and office, like a briefcase or laptop carrier.

P is for: Plantar Warts, Poor Circulation, Poison Ivy and Psoriasis

Plantar Warts (Verrucas)

Plantar Warts (also known as Verrucas) differ from common warts and usually appear as outgrowth lesions on the bottom of the foot. Plantar Warts can be extremely painful as they are pushed inward by the pressure of walking.

The treatment of Plantar Warts is made more difficult because the skin on the bottom of the foot tends to be thicker. Therefore, the use of band aids or duct tape with Planter Warts is more applicable than with other warts.

Massaging with diluted Tea Tree oil can also be helpful. To do this, blend a small amount of olive oil and a few drops of Tea Tree oil and then massage on the Plantar Wart for at least half a minute or so.

Taking foot baths with a few drops of Tea Tree oil added will also help cure Planter Warts. Soak your infected foot for at least 10 minutes. Then dry thoroughly with a fresh clean towel.

To help prevent any type of wart re-occurring, add 4 drops of Tea Tree oil to your bath water.

Poor Circulation

To increase blood circulation to your feet, ankles and legs; add a few drops of Tea Tree oil to an Arnica massage cream and apply vigorously.

Poison Ivy

After a nice day out in the country you come home with an itchy, bubbly rash. If your rash was caused by poison ivy or a similar plant you need to keep the itchiness at bay and get the healing process under way as soon as possible.

Thoroughly wash and dry the affected areas. Use ice to cool the rash if the area isn't too large. Then apply 100% Tea Tree oil directly on the rash and use a Q-tip or a piece of cotton to spread it around. After applying a few times a day the blisters will heal and the rash disappear.

A study by Flinders University showed that the application of 100% Tea Tree oil significantly reduced histamine skin inflammations of the type caused by poison ivy.

Precautions

Used externally Tea Tree oil is considered very safe, but some individuals with sensitive skin may experience an allergic reaction to undiluted Tea Tree oil; causing itchiness, irritation, or redness. When using the oil for the first time, it would be sensible to test it on a very small patch of skin (perhaps under the arm) before applying it to larger areas. If you find your skin is sensitive you can always dilute the oil in water, or in one of many base oils such as olive oil. (Note: base oils are often referred to as carrier oils)

Also, Tea Tree oil should not be ingested without first consulting your medical practitioner.

Always avoid contact with the eyes and keep out of the reach of children!

Remember to tighten the cap after use to avoid oxidation and evaporation. When used and stored properly - tightly sealed and kept away from light and heat - 100% Tea Tree oil does not pose a risk to human health. Correctly formulated products containing Tea Tree oil also pose no risk..

Later in the book I explain when it is OK to use the oil

in its pure form, when and how you should dilute it and which other essential oils you can blend with it.

However don't let these sensible precautions put you off; I and millions of others have used Tea Tree oil without experiencing any adverse effects..

Psoriasis

Make a bath mixture of 5 drops Tea Tree oil, 10 drops Jojoba oil and 1 cup of sea salt. Just dissolve into the bath water for a skin soothing soak.

Or you can dab (not rub) Tea Tree oil directly to your problem areas. After the Tea Tree oil has been absorbed apply an Arnica cream.

R is for: Ringworm

Ringworm

Despite its name, Ringworm is a condition caused by a skin fungus, not worms. It has much in common with Athlete's Foot, Nail Fungus and Jock Itch, and thrives in the same type of conditions. The infection is often spread by skin coming into contact with clothing or towels used by people with one of the above ailments. It is thought that up to 20% of the population may be infected by Ringworm at one time or another.

Tea Tree oil is certainly one of the best remedies for dealing with Ringworm and the process of treating it is very straight forward; just follow these simple steps:

Clean the affected area and it's surrounds with quite a strong dilution; mixing one teaspoon of Tea Tree oil with a half cup of warm water. Ensure the whole area has been treated. (The area can sometimes be quite large) Dry the area and make sure any linens used are put in the dirty laundry to avoid risk of further contamination.

Pour several drops of undiluted Tea Tree oil onto a small piece of sterile cotton gauze and apply it directly to the Ringworm. Make sure all the visible Ringworm has been treated with the oil. If the undiluted oil irritates the skin use the strongest dilution your skin can tolerate.

Repeat this treatment at least three times a day.

It may take several weeks to clear up a severe infection but in any case continue the treatment for some days after the skin has cleared. This will ensure all the infection has gone for good.

S is for: Shaving, Sinus Infection, Slivers and Splinters, Skin Care, Spider Spray, Sprains and Sunburn

Shaving

Apply 100% pure Tea Tree oil directly to small cuts or nicks for quick healing. You can even put a drop on the razor blade to help prevent cuts.

Sinus Infection

If you are one of the millions who regularly suffer a Sinus Infection and you want to become less reliant on antibiotics, you will be pleased to know there is an alternative! Tea Tree oil's anti-bacterial and antiviral properties make it the ideal home remedy for any sort of infection of the nasal and respiratory system.

There are several ways to use Tea Tree oil for Sinus Infection but the most popular way is the 'vapors steaming treatment'. Simply add several drops of Tea Tree oil to boiling water and place a towel over your head to inhale the fumes for 5-10 minutes. This inhalation will loosen phlegm and relieve any pressure or soreness.

This **'vapors steaming treatment'** acts very quickly. Use the treatment once in the morning and again at night.

If nasal congestion is making it difficult for you to sleep at night rub a few drops of the oil on your nose or forehead. Or apply with a cotton bud if you prefer. You can mix with Almond oil if you experience any skin irritation.

I used to add drops of Tea Tree oil to petroleum jelly when my children were poorly and rubbed this on their chest at bedtime. The vapors helped keep their nasal passages clear so they could enjoy a good night's sleep.

Slivers & Splinters

Clean thoroughly with a Tea Tree oil wash and then apply a few drops of undiluted Tea Tree oil. If possible, remove the splinter gently with a needle or tweezers that have been sterilized with Tea Tree oil.

Skin Care

There are many Tea Tree oil skin care products available but you can make your own, by adding a few drops Tea Tree oil to your regular moisturizer.

Spider Spray

For a very effective Spider Spray, just mix 1 teaspoon Tea Tree oil, 2 tablespoons liquid dish soap, and 2 cups of water together in a spray bottle. I use this spray under my wicker furniture in the sunroom and under the plastic chairs that we occasional use on the outside porch, but you can use it anywhere you have a problem with spiders - which reminds me, I need to spray at the back of the storage containers in the garage!

Also works well on ant runs.

Sprains

Arnica Montana is the best remedy for sprains, but Tea Tree oil can be very helpful.

First apply ice to reduce the swelling and then add a few drops of Tea Tree oil to an Arnica gel and apply to the sprain. Bandage the area and, in the case of a sprained ankle, try to keep the foot elevated. Repeat the treatment often.

Sunburn

Add Tea Tree oil to your favorite Coconut oil and spread freely over the affected areas.

Vitamin E, Aloe Vera or Arnica creams can also be mixed with Tea Tree oil to ease sunburn and prevent peeling. The Arnica will reduce inflammation and ease the pain; the Aloe oil will moisturize and the Tea Tree oil, together with Vitamin E will help repair the skin.

In severe cases of sunburn you can apply undiluted Tea Tree oil.

T is for: Tea Tree Sanitizing Wipes and Tired Feet

Tea Tree Sanitizing Wipes

There are literally hundreds of uses for Tea Tree Sanitizing Wipes and dozens of different products on the market. Many of these products make the wipes for particular circumstances i.e. baby wipes, sports wipes, bathroom wipes, facial wipes, etc. I list some of my favorite products below. However, it is relatively easy (and certainly cheaper) to make your own general purpose Tea Tree oil wipes.

There are lots of how-to's on the web and YouTube using everything from paper toweling to old t-shirts. My own favorite is to use coffee filters; they are so versatile they can be used to clean just about anything.

What you need is an old wet wipe container or

something similar. Freezer bags that can zip closed are also viable. I use the larger type coffee filters although any size will suffice. Make a mixture of about 10 drops of Tea Tree oil with one small cup of water - you can experiment with different strengths of this mixture depending on your intended purpose. You could also add a few drops of eucalyptus or lavender oil - my friend Sally adds rubbing alcohol which she finds strengthens the cleaning aspect - but for germ killing, just Tea Tree oil will work fine.

Anyway, once you have your preferred mixture (and please do experiment to find one you really like) place a number of coffee filters in your chosen container and lay them flat to make them easier to pull out when needed. Once you have the coffee filters in place, take the mixture you prepared and pour onto the coffee filters until the bottom coffee filter is saturated. The rest of the coffee filters will quickly soak up the liquid.

My book explains just some of their many potential uses.

Tired Feet

Five drops of Tea Tree oil and a half cup of sea salt (or Epsom salts) in hot water makes a wonderful foot soak. After drying, massage with an Arnica gel and you will soothe your tired feet and feel completely relaxed.

U is for: Unpleasant Smells

Unpleasant Smells

Mix 1 teaspoon of Tea Tree oil with 1 cup of water and use it as a spray to neutralize unpleasant smells around the home. It is marvelous for removing bad odors from practically anything. I like to add a few drops of Lavender to this mixture, especially for a nice bathroom spray.

My son bought a second-hand car which had obviously been owned by a very heavy smoker. It smelled badly of stale cigarette smoke. I really find it difficult to tolerate cigarette smoke at the best of times and the first time I got into his car I got a terrible headache. I sprayed a Tea Tree oil mixture all around the interior of the car and as soon as it dried there was no trace left of cigarette smoke!

Use the same mixture as a room spray to deodorize a smoke filled room. You can also spray clothes to remove cigarette odors.

Tea Tree oil will also remove old food smells from refrigerators and food coolers, and keep them smelling fresh.

Only recently I left a pot on the stove for far too long, but fortunately burned food odor is quickly removed by spraying diluted Tea Tree oil in the room area.

Spray your pet mat or litter boxes to keep them smelling fresh. I often use my husband's car to take my dogs to the local park for their exercise. When we get home, a quick spray with a TeaTree oil mixture removes any lingering 'wet doggy' smells.

V is for Vaginal Thrush

Vaginal Thrush

As mentioned in other chapters of the book, one of Tea Tree oils greatest strengths is as an Anti-fungal agent. Various studies have shown that Tea Tree oil inhibits and kills yeasts, and other fungi. The studies note its particular effectiveness against the Candida Albicans yeast, a common cause of vaginal thrush.

Mix 6 drops of Tea Tree oil in one cup of purified water and soak a tampon in this solution before inserting in the vagina. The tampon should be changed every 24 hours.

W is for: Warts and Waxing

Warts

Warts can be frustratingly difficult to get rid of and there seems to be no perfect treatment for them. They occur pretty much anywhere on the body and can be contagious. Medical treatment consists of over-the-counter medications, freezing the Wart with liquid nitrogen, burning with acid or cutting them out. None of the methods prevent the possibility of the Wart coming back.

Even with natural remedies like Tea Tree oil, (which is far more effective than most) the efficacy of the treatment and the time it takes for a wart to disappear can vary from person to person.

My advice is to be patient and just keep going with a Tea Tree oil treatment. Apply it every day until the Warts disappear and take sensible precautions to prevent them returning.

Some people like to cover the Warts with a waterproof Band-Aid after applying Tea Tree oil, while others use duct tape. By all means experiment to find what works best for you.

My recommendation is to use a cotton bud and apply undiluted Tea Tree oil directly on the Wart and let it dry. It's best to do this at night before you go to bed. Remember, Tea Tree oil is super-potent and can irritate the surrounding skin, so coat the surrounding area with petroleum jelly to prevent this.

To help prevent any type of Wart re-occurring, add 4 drops of Tea Tree oil to your bath water.

Waxing

Tea Tree oil is a must for both pre and post waxing. Applying before maximizes wax adhesion and eliminates bacteria; applying post-wax reduces skin irritation. By using Tea Tree oil you also avoid waxing bumps and ingrown hairs.

Use Tea Tree Sanitizing Wipes over the whole area to be waxed prior to waxing. Allow a moment or two to let the oil absorb.

For an upper lip wax it is important cleanse the area with Tea Tree Sanitizing Wipes to remove any dirt or makeup. After cleansing, use a cotton bud to apply a thin layer of undiluted Tea Tree oil.

After waxing apply a Tea Tree moisturizer several times a day until the waxing area has calmed down.

Y is for: Yoga Mats

Yoga Mats

Yoga Mats need to be cleaned after every use and Tea Tree oil is the only cleaner you will need.

1 cup water, 1 tablespoon Cider vinegar and 6 drops of Tea Tree oil - add to an old spray bottle and you have the perfect yoga mat cleaner. Some of my friends add a few drops of lavender.

Spraying your entire mat after every yoga session will ensure that your mat never gets too filthy.

The History of Tea Tree Oil

Tea Tree oil is a natural anti-bacterial disinfectant that is derived from the leaves of the Melaleuca tree.

The tree is native to Australia and has been used by the aboriginal tribes there for thousands of years to heal skin cuts, burns, and infections.

In those days oil was produced by steaming Tea Tree leaves and then squeezing the residue from the leaves and processing it into oil. This oil was then used in a variety of ways to heal a whole range of ailments. Even rubbing crushed leaves on the skin was found to be a useful antiseptic.

Use of Tea Tree oil only became common practice after Arthur Penfold (researcher & chemist) published the first reports of the oil's healing properties in a series of papers in 1932. He rated Tea Tree oil as being over ten times more active than Phenol. (Phenol was once the standard antiseptic used to control surgical infections)

Demand for the oil grew when scientific journals began publishing glowing reports of his clinical trials and this resulted in the establishment of the first commercial production. By then the hand cut plant material was distilled in makeshift, wood-fired bush stills.

In the Second World War, Australian troops were issued with Tea Tree oil as part of their medical kit. The troops found the oil to be so useful in treating tropical infections and infected wounds that, after the war, it became Australia's best known natural remedy.

Sadly, this amazing natural medicine was forgotten for almost 30 years as cheap, synthetic antibiotics flooded the world's medicine markets. The Tea Tree industry was in a state of collapse by the 1960's and the oil became a rare commodity.

Fortunately however, in 1976, Eric White a movie cameraman became seriously interested in the plant after his stepson Chris Dean had a serious foot infection cured by the oil. Eric invested in his own plantation in northern New South Wales. Chris Dean, realizing the commercial potential of his stepfather's project, became the latter-day pioneer of the Australian Tea Tree industry.

Today large cultivated plantations have been formed throughout Western Australia where Tea Tree oil is distilled under controlled conditions. After harvesting, the plant is chipped into small fragments and the oil is extracted by steam distillation. This produces pale yellow oil with a scent similar to that of nutmeg.

Studies

In the study *A comparative study of tea-tree oil versus benzoylperoxide in the treatment of acne*. Researchers Bassett IB, Pannowitz DL, Barnetson RS. wrote:

"Tea-tree oil (an essential oil of the Australian native tree Melaleuca alternifolia) has long been regarded as a useful topical antiseptic agent in Australia and has been shown to have a variety of antimicrobial activities; however, only anecdotal evidence exists for its efficacy in the treatment of various skin conditions. We have performed a single-blind, randomized clinical trial on 124 patients to evaluate the efficacy and skin tolerance of 5% tea-tree oil gel in the treatment of mild to moderate acne when compared with 5% benzoyl peroxide lotion. The results of this study showed that both 5% tea-tree oil and 5% benzoyl peroxide had a significant effect in ameliorating the patients' acne by reducing the number of inflamed and non-inflamed lesions (open and closed comedones), although the onset of action in the case of tea-tree oil was slower. Encouragingly, fewer side effects were experienced by patients treated with tea-tree oil."
J Am Acad Dermatol. 2002 Dec;47(6):852-5.

In the study *'Treatment of dandruff with 5% Tea Tree oil shampoo'*.Satchell AC, Saurajen A, Bell C, Barnetson RS.

Source;Department of Dermatology, Royal Prince Alfred Hospital, Camperdown, NSW, Australia.

Abstract; BACKGROUND: Dandruff appears to be related to the yeast Pityrosporum ovale. Tea Tree oil has anti-fungal properties with activity against P ovale and may be useful in the treatment of dandruff.

OBJECTIVE: We conducted a randomized, single-blind, parallel-group study to investigate the efficacy and tolerability of 5% Tea Tree oil and placebo in patients with mild to moderate dandruff.

METHODS: One hundred twenty-six male and female patients, aged 14 years and older, were randomly assigned to receive either 5% Tea Tree oil shampoo or placebo, which was used daily for 4 weeks. The dandruff was scored on a quadrant-area-severity scale and by patient self-assessment scores of scaliness, itchiness, and greasiness.

RESULTS: The 5% Tea Tree oil shampoo group showed a 41% improvement in the quadrant-area-severity score compared with 11% in the placebo group ($P < .001$). Statistically significant improvements were also observed in the total area of involvement score, the total severity score, and the itchiness and greasiness components of the patients' self-assessments. The scaliness component of patient self-assessment improved but was not statistically significant. There were no adverse effects.

CONCLUSION: Five percent Tea Tree oil appears to effective and well tolerated in the treatment of dandruff.

PMID:12451368 [PubMed - indexed for MEDLINE]

Message from the Author

Thank you so much for reading my book; I do hope you found it interesting and helpful.

My publishers have called this 'A Complete Guide', but of course there is no such thing as 'complete' when it comes to the uses of Tea Tree oil. It seems like almost everyday, I receive a story from someone who has found yet another way to successfully use the oil to help with an ailment or to put it to some other practical use.

It is my ambition to build up an overwhelming body of anecdotal evidence in support of the healing properties of Tea Tree oil and I would love to hear your story.

Anecdotal evidence is how most knowledge has been developed throughout history. How best to do anything was figured out by seeing what worked, and then passing that information to others. People learned that certain herbs had curative value by first trying and then handing their experiences down through generations, as anecdotal evidence.

I believe the medical testimony of others truly counts as evidence and I would really like to know your experience of Tea Tree oil. Not just positive experiences; I would even like to know in what circumstances Tea Tree oil didn't work for you or caused side effects.

I hope you agree that all experiences, from the widest source possible, will provide valuable information on which others can base health decisions. If you do, please share yours.

If you have an anecdote about Tea Tree oil you would like to share, please help me by sending it to: tto.mystory@gmail.com.

Thank you!

Best wishes in health!

Ruth Elston 2013

References

Altman, P. M. 1988. Australian Tea Tree oil. Aust. J. Pharm. 69:276-278

Bassett, I. B., D. L. Pannowitz, and R. S. Barnetson. 1990. A comparative study of tea-tree oil versus benzoylperoxide in the treatment of acne. Med. J. Aust. 153:455-458. [PubMed]

Bischoff, K., and F. Guale. 1998. Australian Tea Tree (Melaleuca alternifolia) oil poisoning in three purebred cats. J. Vet. Diagn. Investig. 10:208-210. [PubMed]

Blackwell, R. 1991. An insight into aromatic oils: lavender and Tea Tree. Br. J. Phytother. 2:26-30.

Buck, D.S D. M. Nidorf, and J.G. Addino, Treatment of Nail Fungus: A Comparison of Two Topical Preparations. Journal of Family Practice, June; 38(6): 601-5 1994 Carson, C. F., and T. V. Riley. 1993. Antimicrobial activity of the essential oil of Melaleuca alternifolia. Lett. Appl. Microbiol. 16:49-55.

Discovery Health "Repelling Mosquitoes Naturally"

EFFECTIVENESS AND SAFETY OF AUSTRALIAN TEA TREE OIL, THE © 2007 Rural Industries Research and Development Corporation ISBN 1 74151 539 4 Publication No. 07/143

Finlay-Jones J, Hart P, Riley T, Carson C (2001). Anti-inflammatory activity of Tea Tree oil. RIRDC Report #01/10.

Hammer K, Carson C, Riley, T (2002). Anti-fungal activity of Tea Tree oil. Project UWA-58A. Rural Industries Research and Development Corporation

Health911.com Nail Infections - - Toe Nail Fungus, Fungus in Nail Low, T. 1990. Bush medicine. Harper Collins Publishers, North Ryde, NSW, Australia

Maruzzella, J. C., and N. A. Sicurella. 1960. Anti-bacterial activity of essential oil vapors. J. Am. Pharm. Assoc. 49:692-694Penfold,A.R., and F.R. Morrison. "Some Notes on the Essential Oil of Melaleuca alternifolia." British Medical Journal, 1933.

PubMed: Abstract: Australasian Journal of Dermatology: Treatment of Interdigital Tinea Pedis with 25 and 50 Percent Tea Tree Oil Solution

Richter, Allan Natural Treasures of Australia. Energy Times May 2012

Rushton, R. T., N. W. Davis, J. C. Page, and C. A. Durkin. 1997. The effect of Tea Tree oil extract on the growth of fungi. Lower Extremity 4:113-116

Satchell, A. C., A. Saurajen, C. Bell, and R. S. Barnetson. 2002. Treatment of dandruff with 5% Tea Tree oil shampoo. J. Am. Acad. Dermatol. 47:852-855. [PubMed]

Teicher, Shayna - Tea Tree Oil vs. Ringworm | Modern Hippie Mag June 9, 2010

Tong, M. M., P. M. Altman, and R. S. Barnetson. 1992. Tea Tree oil in the treatment of tinea pedis. Aust. J. Dermatol. 33:145-149.

Urich P Saxer. Effect of mouthwashing with Tea Tree oil on plaque and inflammation. Prophylaxe Zentrum Zürich, Klinikleiter Lehrbeauftragter für Parodontologie und Präventivzahnmedizin, Universität Zürich Zentrum für Zahn, Switzerland Schweiz Monatsschr Zahnmed 113:985-96. 2003

Walker, M. 1972. Clinical investigation of Australian Melaleuca alternifolia oil for a variety of common foot problems. Curr. Podiatry 1972:7-15.

Weil, Dr. Andrew Treating Ringworm With Tea Tree Oil

Wikipedia, the free encyclopedia - Tea Tree oil

www.dailymail.co.uk/health/article-4018/The-wonders-Tea-Tree-oil

Disclaimer

The information contained in this guide is not presented by a medical practitioner and is not designed to replace or take the place of any form of medicine or professional medical advice. You should consult your doctor, veterinarian or get other professional medical advice before using any of the suggested remedies in this guide.

This guide has been provided for educational and informative purposes only. All links in this report are for information purposes only and are not warranted for content, accuracy or any other implied or explicit purpose.

In self-help books, as in life, there are no guarantees of results. Readers are cautioned to rely on their own good judgment about their individual circumstances and act accordingly.

Printed in Great Britain
by Amazon.co.uk, Ltd.,
Marston Gate.